A FISHY FUTURE

The omega-3 fatty acids EPA and DHA, found in cold-water fish, are producing a near-revolution in approaches to such conditions as heart disease, arthritis, diabetes, migraines and some forms of cancer. Definitive research is still being done, and the most exciting discoveries are yet to come, but the work surveyed here indicates strongly that good health and substantial fish intake are closely linked.

ABOUT THE AUTHOR AND EDITORS

Richard A. Passwater, Ph.D. is one of the most called-upon authorities for information relating to preventive health care. A noted biochemist, he is credited with popularizing the term "supernutrition," largely as a result of having written two bestsellers on the subject—*Supernutrition: Megavitamin Revolution* and *Supernutrition for Healthy Hearts*. His other books include *Easy No-Flab Diet, Cancer and Its Nutritional Therapies, Selenium as Food & Medicine, Hair Analysis and Nutrition* (with Elmer M. Cranton, M.D.) and The Good Health Guides *Selenium Update* and *Fish Oils Update*.

Earl Mindell, R.Ph., Ph.D. combines the expertise and working experience of a pharmacist with extensive knowledge in most of the nutrition areas. *Earl Mindell's Vitamin Bible* and *Vitamin Bible for Your Kids* are major bestsellers; his latest book is *Unsafe at Any Meal*. Dr. Mindell's popular *Quick & Easy Guide to Better Health* is published by Keats Publishing, as is *The Vitamin Robbers*, a Good Health Guide.

FISH OILS UPDATE

LATEST RESEARCH ON MARINE LIPIDS AND THEIR NEWLY DISCOVERED HEALTH ROLES

by Richard A. Passwater, Ph.D.

Keats Publishing Inc.   New Canaan, Connecticut

Fish Oils Update is not intended as medical advice. Its intention is solely informational and educational. Please consult a medical or health professional should the need for one be indicated.

FISH OILS UPDATE

ISBN: 0-87983-432-3

Printed in the United States of America

Good Health Guides are published by
Keats Publishing, Inc.
27 Pine Street (Box 876)
New Canaan, Connecticut 06840

Contents

The amazing benefits of fish oils continue to be discovered by today's medical researchers. In 1982, when I wrote the Good Health Guide *EPA—Marine Lipids*,[1] the research indicated that fish oils could dramatically reduce heart disease, but the biochemistry concerning the interrelationships of fish oils, prostaglandins and health were so unknown to nutritionists and physicians that I had to devote much of the booklet to explaining the biochemistry involved.

Now fish oils are so widely recognized for their beneficial role in preventing and/or alleviating heart disease, high blood pressure, arthritis and migraine headaches that there is barely room to discuss these new studies in this book. In addition, there is exciting research that shows that fish oils may be protective against cancer, immune deficiency diseases, kidney disease and others. So, in this Good Health Guide, I will concentrate on practical health information.

On the very day that I gathered my notes to compile this update, there were several articles in the *New England Journal of Medicine* extolling the many benefits of fish oils, plus a front-page story in *USA Today* telling of still one more way in which fish oils protect the heart.

The new knowledge involving the balancing of dietary oils to optimize prostaglandin production undoubtedly will lead to many more beneficial health discoveries in the near future. Therefore, I'll give a brief review of basics here, but those wanting more details about how fish oils make prostaglandins and how prostaglandins work to restore health can consult Reference 1.

Fish oils are of such great importance because they contain two special nutrients. These special nutrients form the compounds that protect the heart and arteries, reduce pain, inflammation and swelling and protect cell membranes. Strangely enough, these special nutrients belong to the *fat* family of nutrients. In spite of the fact that many people have too much fat overall in their diet, most people are lacking these special fats or they can't produce sufficient quantities of them from other dietary fats. Many researchers believe that most people are getting too much of the wrong kinds of fats, and need the fish oil fats to *balance* the family of fat nutrients.

Most people's diets have too many animal-source saturated fats and too many vegetable-source polyunsaturated fats, and should lower total fat intake to 20 to 30 percent of daily calorie intake, while appreciably increasing intake of the fats found in the oils of certain fish. In addition, a significant number of people will benefit from increasing the amount of still another fat called gamma-linolenic acid (GLA).*

The point is that fat is not fat is not fat! Just as there are different vitamins and different amino acids, with each having their own metabolic tasks, there are different fats which have different body functions. We have learned not to think only in terms of vitamin A and protein, but in terms of a balance of all vitamins and amino acids. Now we should learn to think in terms of a balance of all fat groups.

*Gamma-linolenic acid is an important fatty acid found in human milk, evening primrose oil, black currants, borage oil and a few other foods. The importance of GLA to nutrition and health is discussed in my Good Health Guide *Evening Primrose Oil.*

As an example of the effect of different fats on health and lifespan, consider the study by Dr. A. Bennett at Ball State University in Muncie, Indiana.[2] Mice were fed a high-fat diet rich in either the polyunsaturated fatty acid linoleic acid, the primary fat in vegetable oils, or the saturated fatty acid stearic acid, the primary fat in beef. The average lifespan of mice fed the linoleic acid-rich diet was less than 20 months, while the average lifespan of mice fed the saturated fat was more than 30 months. No, that's not a typo, the mice lived more than 50 percent longer on the saturated animal fat diet than on the polyunsaturates. Yet many people are being urged to eat more polyunsaturated, rather than saturated fats.

The significant point is that fats are different and different dietary fats may have varying effects on health and lifespan.

Oils and fats are both members of the same chemical family called lipids. Actually the word "fat" is an acceptable word for non-chemists to use in place of "lipid." It is also acceptable to call lipids that are solid at room temperature fats, and lipids that are liquid at room temperature oils.

The number of atoms in each molecule and the degree of saturation of each molecule help to determine whether a lipid is solid or liquid at room temperature.

Fish oils and vegetable oils are both made up of largely polyunsaturated fatty acids (PUFA). Fatty acids are the basic units of fats. Typical body fats are formed by joining three fatty acids to a frame of glycerol. Basically, there are two major families of PUFA: the omega-6 (ω-6 or n-6) family and the omega-3 (ω-3 or n-3) family; and one major family of monounsaturated fatty acids, the omega-9 (ω-9 or n-9). The difference between the families is in the position of the double bonds. In omega-3 fats, the first double bond is three carbon atoms from the terminal end (omega) of the molecule; in omega-6 fats, it's six carbon atoms, and so on. Chemists consider the methyl group to be the end of the fatty acid molecule and the carboxyl acid group to be the beginning of the molecule.

The major dietary source of the omega-6 family is linoleic acid (LA). In modern Western diets the major source of the omega-3 family is alpha-linolenic acid (ALA). In societies having low incidence of heart disease, the major dietary sources of the omega-3 family are often eicosapentaenoic acid (EPA) and docosahexaenoic acid (DHA). The major source of the omega-9 family is oleic acid.

The major dietary fatty acids can to some extent be converted in the body to other fatty acids that are needed for various functions, particularly the production of prostaglandins (PGs), hormone-like compounds having great biologic influence. PGs are regulators that are manufactured in the cells at the point of use, rather than being produced in a distant gland and having to be transported in the bloodstream to where they will be used.

PGs are not stored, and are quickly inactivated by enzymes. Each tissue makes PGs as needed, if the appropriate fatty acid precursors are present in the tissues in adequate quantities. Some organ systems depend on a balance of PGs which act in opposing ways.

Prostaglandins are so named because the first one was isolated in the prostate gland. They control or influence many body processes, including blood pressure, blood clotting, blood sugar, menstrual cramps, gastrointestinal secretion, fertility, reproduction, immunity, inflammation and pain. These functions are involved in heart disease, arthritis, asthma, migraine headaches, glaucoma, diabetes, cancer and other disorders. Some of the functions are desirable, some are not. Desirable functions are usually controlled by the PGs of the PG1 and PG3 family.

The PG1 family is produced from GLA, while the PG3 family is produced from EPA and DHA. The abundant PG2 family is produced from LA and arachidonic acid (AA), both of vegetable source. PG2s produce some desirable functions, as well as several undesirable functions. LA and AA also produce compounds related to PGs that are not desirable.

The conversion of LA to GLA and the conversion of ALA to EPA or DHA are hindered by the wrong diet, illness and aging. The wrong diet, too little of certain vitamins and minerals, and too much saturated fat block the conversion.

Therefore, many individuals do not have optimal stores

of EPA, DHA and GLA and cannot produce optimal amounts of PG3 and PG1. Their prostaglandin production is unbalanced towards PG2, and they tend to have "sticky" blood, membrane problems, inflammation and other difficulties.

For your information, and not to make a big issue of the various types of PGs, it should be pointed out that there are several family members of PGs within each of the PG1, PG2 and PG3 families. They are designated by another letter, such as an "E" or an "F" following the "PG" and before the number. Scientists have identified more than twenty different PGs. Of these, the members designated as PGEs, PGFs and PGIs are the most important.

This may be more than you ever wanted to know about fatty acids and PGs. It is presented for your information, but you certainly don't have to understand all that chemical jargon to understand the test results and facts about how fish oil protects against all those diseases. It will help you to understand why fish oil works, but we used aspirin for a century before we understood how it worked. (Which, by the way, turns out to be via its influence on PGs.)

The key is a balance of the PGs and the dietary fats. While stressing the importance of EPA, DHA and GLA and emphasizing their disparity in the diet, keep in mind that LA still is an important dietary factor. The daily diet should contain about three grams of LA. As Dr. J. Kinsella points out in *Nutrition Today*, "no other nutrient affects so many physiological interactions as does LA via its conversion to AA and thence to (PG2 and related compounds)."[3] However, Americans average about 25 grams of LA, which far exceeds the requirement and actually becomes a problem because some of the products formed from LA interfere with the conversion to desirable PGs.

That's the background; now let's look at the research findings.

One of the first human studies reported was conducted by Von Lossonczy *et al.* in 1978.[4] He used Cistercian monks and nuns in a three-week cross-over design experiment in which they were given a daily portion of mackerel which is rich in EPA and DHA. During the low omega-3 fatty acid period, cheese was substituted for the mackerel.

During the initial EPA-rich diet period, the volunteers' serum cholesterol and triglyceride levels dropped, but after three weeks on the cheese, these levels had been restored.

Van Gent *et al.* fed groups of ten non-fish eating volunteers a fish oil concentrate containing 81 percent omega-3 acids including 25 percent EPA and 38 percent DHA.[5] They found that at intakes of up to 8 grams per day of omega-3 fatty acids for four weeks, there was no significant change in serum cholesterol or HDL cholesterol. Serum triglycerides and VLDL (very low density level) did, however, fall significantly. The lack of effect on HDL cholesterol may have been due to the possibility that they used an omega-3 supplement based on ethyl esters. Such a form of presentation has been known to show different effects from that given by an omega-3 EPA.[6]

Mackerel was also used in a study by Siess *et al.*[7] These workers fed volunteers for a week on a diet containing 500-800 grams of stewed or smoked mackerel, together with a source of carbohydrate (unspecified). They found a marked change in the clumping, and unwanted stickiness of blood platelets.

Harris and Connor[8] fed salmon oil diets to volunteers for four weeks. The diets were formulated to provide almost half of the calories as fat. On the treatment diet, the fat was omega-3 fatty acids, while the control diet contained no omega-3 fatty acids. They found that after four weeks on the salmon meat/salmon oil diet, their subjects showed significantly lower levels of total cholesterol and serum triglycerides.

Saynor and Verel fed 20 milliliters of EPA, for five weeks to volunteers and found a rise in HDL cholesterol and a fall in serum triglycerides but no significant change in total cholesterol.

Saynor and Verel have extended their original observations to heart patients and found much the same results as in their earlier studies.[9]

A study conducted at the University of Oregon Health Sciences Center, Portland, was reported in the *Journal of the American Medical Association*. Using a ten-day diet of salmon which contains both EPA and DHA, plasma cholesterol levels dropped by 17 percent in presumably healthy volunteers and by 20 percent or more in patients who had elevated cholesterol and mildly elevated triglyceride levels. The triglyceride levels fell as much as 40 percent in healthy volunteers and by as much as 67 percent in those whose levels had been elevated originally.

In *EPA–Marine Lipids*, covering research through mid-1982, I described the epidemiological research that gave scientists the clue that there might be some factor in fish oil that protected the Eskimos from heart disease. Eskimos eat a very high-fat diet and according to conventional wisdom would be expected to have a very high incidence of heart disease instead of their actual very low rate. When Europeans normally eating a Westernized diet were switched to an Eskimo-like diet high in cold-water fish, the European volunteers had changes in their blood that are associated with protection against heart attacks.

Low death rates from heart disease are also found in Japan, where fish intake is very high. Within Japan, the lowest heart disease death rate is found on the island of Okinawa, where fish consumption is about twice as high as on the mainland. In a study in the Chiba Perfecture, residents of fishing villages had lower heart disease death rates than those living in farming villages. Fish consumption in the fishing village averaged about 9 ounces compared to about 3.2 ounces in the farming villages.

Follow-up experiments with fish oil, first in laboratory animals and then in clinical trials, found the same changes in blood chemistry—blood that was more free-flowing or less sticky that tended not to clot as easily. Blood that clots too easily is prone to collect in narrowed coronary arteries and shut off the blood flow to the heart. This is called a heart attack or coronary thrombosis, and results in heart tissue destruction, which is called myocardial infarction.

Other beneficial changes to the blood produced by fish oil noted by the researchers were lowered cholesterol and triglyceride levels.

Laboratory animal experiments continued to broaden our knowledge and add more mechanisms showing how fish oils reduce heart attacks. In November 1982, researchers at the University of Michigan Medical School demonstrated that fish oil decreases the reactivity of blood vessels to stress hormones.[10]

A small-scale clinical study in Japan indicated that EPA reduced TXB2 (a thromboxane that can cause clotting), platelet aggregation (a measure of blood's tendency to clot) and blood viscosity. The researchers concluded that EPA produces no side effects and may be useful in the treatment and prevention of thrombotic diseases—disease involving blood clotting as is the case in most heart attacks.[11]

Cholesterol and triglycerides. The Harris-Connor group examined the effect of fish oil on high-carbohydrate diets. These diets increase the blood levels of very-low-density lipoproteins (VLDL) and triglycerides. VLDL are carriers that transport mostly triglycerides and some cholesterol in the blood. They are smaller than the more familiar low-density lipoproteins (LDL) and high-density lipoproteins (HDL). It is well recognized that having more HDL than LDL protects against heart disease. The role of VLDL is not as well understood, but some researchers feel that high levels of VLDL are also a risk factor in heart disease.

The studies compared the effects of fish oils and plant oils on the blood levels of VLDL and triglycerides in healthy persons eating a high-carbohydrate diet. The healthy volunteers were placed on a diet that was 45 percent carbohydrate and 45 percent fat for a period of time to establish baseline measurements. Next they were placed on a 75 percent carbohydrate diet, 15 percent of which consisted of peanut oil and cocoa butter. (Either that tastes better than I think, or we have here an example of self-sacrifice in the cause of science!) After a period of time, the plant fats were replaced with fish oils, while the remainder of the diet was unchanged.

When the volunteers consumed the high-carbohydrate diet without the fish oils, their blood levels of triglycerides rose an average of 85 percent while their VLDL more than doubled. But when they were switched to the high-carbohydrate diet with fish oils, their blood level of triglycerides dropped from the elevated level to a level that was even lower than the baseline level associated with the moderate-carbohydrate diet. Their average VLDL level dropped 78 percent and the cholesterol level dropped 65 percent to below baseline level. These effects were seen within three days of adding fish oil to the diet.[12,13]

In 1985, members of this research group reported that fish oils produced dramatic drops in blood triglyceride levels in patients having highly elevated levels of these fats. Fish oils were far more effective than corn oil or safflower oil.[14]

A study from Karlovy University in Prague, Czechoslovakia also showed that fish oils reduced high triglycerides. Men with elevated blood levels of triglycerides who were given about 18 ounces of fish daily for three months had reductions in triglyceride levels and improvements in HDL levels.[15]

In 1986, Dr. Paul Nestel of the Baker Medical Research Institute in Melbourne, Australia showed that adding fish oil to a high-cholesterol diet prevented increased blood cholesterol levels and possibly reduced the risk of heart disease. He fed volunteers three different diets over a seven-week period: a normal diet, a fish-oil diet, and a fish oil–egg yolk diet.

The normal diet had a PUFA-to-saturated fat ratio of 0.47 and a daily cholesterol level of 710 milligrams. The fish oil diet (40 grams of MaxEPA per day) had a PUFA-to-saturated fat ratio of 1.62 and a daily cholesterol level of 190 milligrams. The fish oil–egg yolk diet had a PUFA-to-saturated fat ratio of 1.62 and a daily cholesterol level of 940 milligrams.

When the volunteers were switched from the normal diet to the fish oil diet, their blood cholesterol, VLDL, LDL, HDL and triglyceride levels declined. When they were then switched to the fish oil–egg yolk (high cholesterol) diet, the expected elevation in those blood components did not occur, however, cholesterol levels did rise slightly. It was concluded that fish oils are effective in lowering lipoprotein cholesterol levels even when the dietary intake of cholesterol is high.[16]

Following up on the laboratory findings reported in 1983, two studies confirmed that fish oils increase the time required for a blood clot to form by reducing the stickiness of the blood platelets that start the clotting mechanism in man as well as in laboratory animals.[17,18]

Coronary mortality. The studies of blood cholesterol and triglycerides are interesting, but do they really mean anything in terms of actual reduction in heart disease or is it just so much theory? To answer that question absolutely, long-term clinical trials are required. However, long-term retrospective studies and short-term prospective clinical trials are available and show significant evidence.

A series of articles and an editorial in the highly respected *New England Journal of Medicine* opened many eyes. Fish oils came of age on May 9, 1985 when these articles were published and were read by doctors who had not even heard of this research until then. One of the articles has already been discussed, but it applied only to the levels of blood components believed to be involved in the heart disease process. The real attention-grabber was an article from the Netherlands.

A research team at the University of Leiden's Institute of Social Medicine in the Netherlands, led by Dr. Daan Kromhout, produced the first long-term study of the effects of fish oils on heart disease deaths.

We were aware of the low death rate from coronary heart disease among the Greenland Eskimos. We therefore decided to investigate the relation between fish consumption and coronary heart disease in a group of men in the town of Zutphen, the Netherlands. Information about the fish consumption of 852 middle-aged men without clinical signs or any other indication of coronary heart disease was collected in 1960 by a careful dietary history obtained from the participants and their wives.

During twenty years of follow-up, 78 men died from coronary heart disease. An inverse dose-response relation was observed between the consumption in 1960 and the death from coronary heart disease during twenty years of follow-up.

This relation persisted after factoring for other variables. Mortality from coronary heart disease was 58 percent lower among those who consumed at least 30 grams (slightly more than an ounce) of fish per day than among those who did not eat fish.

We conclude that the consumption of as little as one or two fish dishes per week may be of preventive value in relation to coronary heart disease.[19]

The relationship existed throughout the time period. Twenty-seven men died from coronary heart disease between 1960 and 1970, 51 between 1971 and 1980. The more fish the men ate, the fewer deaths due to heart disease, and the lower the total death rate, as other diseases were not affected.

For those who worry too much about dietary cholesterol, it should be noted that the men eating the most fish also ate the most cholesterol and animal protein, yet had lower heart disease deaths. Please keep in mind the studies showing that fish and fish oils both tend to lower blood cholesterol levels, regardless of the dietary cholesterol content.

On September 26, 1985, *NEJM* published some of the letters it had received commenting on the three articles and the editorial in the May 9 issue. Among the responses was data from the group that conducted the Western Electric study on heart disease that began in 1957. When Drs. Jeremiah Stamler, Richard Shekelle, Oglesby Paul and their colleagues examined their data in terms of fish consumption versus heart disease death rate, they confirmed the Kromhout group's observations. The Western Electric data showed that the 25-year risk of death from coronary heart disease for those men consuming more than 35 grams of fish per day was only 65 percent of that for those who did not eat fish.[20]

Researchers led by Dr. Robert Wissler of the University of Chicago studied the effects of fish oil on the walls of arteries. They found that fish oil reduced plaque formation in rhesus monkeys, which have arteries and a biochemistry very similar to humans.

The researchers fed 16 rhesus monkeys a diet high in

fish oil, and fed a group of 8 rhesus monkeys a diet similar except that it was high in saturated fat. The monkeys fed the fish oil diet not only developed fewer deposits in their arteries, but the deposits contained fewer inflammatory cells and were less likely to cause medical complications, according to Dr. Wissler. The monkeys fed the fish oil diet had lower blood levels of LDL cholesterol as well.[21]

And just when we think that we have learned all the ways in which fish oils protect us against death by heart attack, another one turns up! Dr. Carl Hock at the University of Medicine and Dentistry of New Jersey told researchers attending the 1986 annual meeting of the American Heart Association of experiments in which he fed a group of laboratory rats a diet with the predominant fat being fish oils and another group a diet with corn oil predominating.[22] After four weeks, he blocked the flow of blood to the rats' hearts. The rats that were fed fish oils had less tissue damage and less loss of an important enzyme usually destroyed during a heart attack.

He also found that EPA had become part of the heart's cell structure.

We have seen that fish oils reduce the heart disease death rate in people over periods of from 10 to 25 years, that fish oils reduce the development of coronary artery disease and protect the heart against damage from heart attack. It was also reassuring to note that fish oils reduced the blood levels of factors that are associated with the risk of heart disease. But there is still more to the story.

Blood Pressure. High blood pressure is called a "silent killer" because it produces no pain or symptoms, yet it is a major risk factor for stroke and other diseases of the arteries. The good news is that fish oils, at least some of them, help normalize blood pressure.

Physicians at the Central Institute for Cardiovascular Research in the German Democratic Republic reported in July 1985 that a mackerel diet containing 2.2 grams of EPA daily produced a significantly lower systolic (upper number) blood pressure in eight of eight patients having an inherited disorder that produces abnormally high blood triglyceride and cholesterol levels and premature heart disease. The disease is called familial hyperlipoproteinemia. The mackerel diet also reduced blood cholesterol and triglycerides for a period of three months, after which they tended to drift back towards their previous values, as is the usual case with these patients and dietary modification.[23]

Later this research group studied 14 patients having moderate high blood pressure (essential hypertension). The mackerel diet decreased systolic blood pressure by almost 10 percent. Whenever the subjects were returned to their normal diets, their blood pressure increased again. When they were again given the mackerel diet, their blood pressure dropped towards normal.

Other blood parameters associated with high blood pressure were also improved. Blood sodium (salt) levels decreased and renin (a hormone produced in the kidney that greatly affects blood pressure) activity increased by 64 percent. The researchers concluded that these data suggest a beneficial effect of a mackerel diet on patients with mild essential hypertension.[24]

In 1986, researchers at the London Chest Hospital studied 16 patients having mild hypertension. They were given MaxEPA fish oil capsules for 12 weeks in a placebo controlled, cross-over study. Their blood pressure averaged 160/94 at the start of the study. After being on a placebo for six weeks, their blood pressures remained at an average of 161/94.5 as would be expected. However, after being switched to MaxEPA fish oil capsules for six weeks, their blood pressures dropped to an average of 151/92.5. The drop in systolic pressure was statistically significant.

Most patients reported that they preferred the fish oil supplements to their previous treatment. The researchers concluded that fish oil supplementation may provide a safe, more acceptable treatment for patients with mild essential systolic hypertension who are reluctant to embark on drug therapies.[25]

Heart disease is what aroused scientific interest in fish oils, but now that we are beginning to understand the biochemistry involved we are seeing that EPA can bring benefit to a host of health problems.

Arthritis and lupus. Animal studies at Harvard indicated that EPA helps protect the body against attack by its own immune system in autoimmune diseases such as rheumatoid arthritis and lupus erythematosus.[27,28]

The researchers were studying the effects of EPA on the inflammatory process and kidney disease. They reasoned that, if EPA reduces the body's production of inflammatory compounds, it should aid arthritis and lupus sufferers. A key factor in the inflammation process is leukotriene B4 (LTB4). LTB4 can make a major contribution to joint discomfort and pain. Tissues can make LTB4 out of omega-6 fatty acids, but when omega-3 fatty acid EPA is present, leukotriene B5 (LTB5) is made instead. LTB5 is relatively benign in comparison to LTB4.

A 1985 article in *Clinical Research* reported that fish oil supplements significantly improved the health of rheumatoid arthritis patients. Dr. Joel M. Kremer, an associate professor of medicine at Albany Medical College, and his colleagues reported a 40-patient, placebo-controlled, double-blind, cross-over study.[29] They gave 15 MaxEPA capsules daily to 20 patients for 14 weeks. The patients continued their normal diets with the only difference being the MaxEPA supplement. At the same time another group of 20 arthritis patients took the same number of placebo capsules.

After the 14-week period, all 40 patients began a 4-week

washout period in which they took no MaxEPA or placebo. The groups were then "cross-overed," i.e., each group then took the capsules formerly taken by the other group, for 14 weeks. Another 4-week washout period followed. Thirty-three patients completed the clinical trial. Dr. Kremer reports, "Those taking fish oil had only about half the number of tender joints as they had prior to the study, and about half as many as the patients taking the placebo. The benefit vanished during the washout period." The researchers also noted that MaxEPA slowed the onset of fatigue.

Dr. Kremer also gave an updated report on the study at the 1986 annual meeting of the American Rheumatism Association (ARA), in which he reported that MaxEPA produced a 60 percent reduction in LTB4 in humans as well as laboratory animals, and increased the production of LTB5 in humans. Dr. Kremer reported, "We saw a significant correlation between the drop in leukotriene B4 and the decrease in the number of tender joints. Those receiving the EPA supplement weren't in as much pain, their joints were less tender and they made it through the day longer before fatigue set in."

Dr. Dwight R. Robinson, a rheumatologist at Massachusetts General Hospital, reported that MaxEPA has the most striking protective effect seen thus far in any animal tests of inflammatory diseases. He found that MaxEPA was effective in laboratory mice having systemic lupus. The National Institutes of Health conducted a multicentered study of about 60 systemic lupus patients and is preparing to report their results at the time of this writing.

Migraines. And the fish oil story goes on. There is even good news for migraineurs—migraine sufferers.

Fish oil dramatically reduces the frequency and severity of migraine headaches, according to studies at the University of Cincinnati Medical Center. Dr. Charles J. Glueck and his associates conducted a 19-week, double-blind, placebo-crossover controlled, clinical trial involving 8 women and 7 men, were severe classic migraineurs who had not responded to any of the gamut of antimigraine therapy that they received. They were given either

15 grams of MaxEPA or placebo for six weeks, followed by a three-week placebo washout period, and then "crossed over" for six weeks to the opposite formulation.[29]

In males, MaxEPA significantly reduced migraines. In females, there was no significant difference between MaxEPA and the placebo. There was a significant reduction in headaches for the entire group. Five of the seven men had a greater than 33 percent reduction in headache score, while only two of eight women had a reduction in excess of 33 percent.

The researchers concluded that "the migraine ameliorating action of MaxEPA may be mediated through changes in prostaglandin synthesis and/or by reductions in platelet serotonin release, with an aggregate diminution in cerebral vasospasm." The researchers noted that nutritional supplementation with fish oil is a promising way to relieve migraine pain. It can benefit migraineurs who have not responded to drug therapy, who don't like to take medication, or who have severe reactions to migraine medications.

Cancer. Research also suggests that diets high in fish oils may help prevent and arrest growth of breast, colon, prostate and pancreatic cancers. Dr. Rashida Karmali of Rutgers University and Memorial Sloan-Kettering Hospital has found that fish oil counteracts the action of vegetable oils that promote harmful cell changes.

In Dr. Karmali's studies, which were reported to the 1986 annual meeting of the American Dietetic Association in Las Vegas, rats given corn oil were compared to those given corn oil plus fish oil. Those given the fish oil had significantly fewer and smaller breast tumors. Dr. Karmali's colon and prostate experiments also indicate that fish oil is protective against those cancers.

In an earlier study, Dr. Karmali's group had shown that EPA inhibited the growth of transplanted tumors (mammary adenocarcinoma). MaxEPA was given orally to laboratory rats for one week before and three weeks after they received the transplants of cancer tissue. The laboratory animals were maintained on standard laboratory diets, with the exception that different groups were given different amounts of EPA. After three weeks, tumor growth was significantly less in the three MaxEPA groups than in the unsupplemented controls.

Levels of AA were higher in tumors from laboratory animals given MaxEPA, and levels of prostaglandin and thromboxane products of AA metabolism were reduced. Tumor microsomes from animals given MaxEPA had decreased ability to synthesize AA metabolites. The researchers concluded that inhibition of AA metabolism may be a mammary cancer-reducing mechanism.[30]

In a study at Cornell University, rats injected with a chemical known to cause pancreatic cancer had fewer and smaller tumors with fish oil than with corn oil.[31] Dr. T. P. O'Connor and his colleagues concluded that, "this study provides evidence that fish oils, rich in omega-3 fatty acids, may have potential as inhibitory agents in cancer development."

In a similar experiment, fish oil again proved to be an effective protector against cancer. Drs. J. Jurkowski and W. Cave of St. Mary's Hospital in Rochester used menhaden fish oil as the EPA source and N-methyl-N-nitrosourea as the cancer-causing chemical. The laboratory rats given fish oil survived an average of 38 percent longer, had 75 percent fewer tumors, and total tumor mass was 80 percent less than those not getting the fish oil.

All animals on their normal diets developed cancer, whereas 37.5 percent of rats given fish oil remained free of cancer. When corn oil was added to the normal diets, there was no significant change, and all of the rats developed cancer. Analysis of relevant tissues confirmed that EPA levels were inversely related to tumor development.[32]

It is thus apparent that cancer protection is a function of prostaglandin balance, not polyunsaturation. In fact, polyunsaturation from the omega-6 family—the LA from corn oil and other vegetable oils—is suspected of being a contributor to cancer development when the omega-6 PUFAs become excessive. Antioxidants such as vitamins A, C and E, plus the trace mineral selenium, are needed to counteract the excess of vegetable oils in today's diets. The cancer rate would drop dramatically if, on the average, vegetable oil consumption (but not whole vegetables) would drop, antioxidant nutrient consumption would increase, and EPA intake would increase.

If you are still unconvinced that the difference in the PUFA family and balance of PGs are not critical factors in cancer development, consider the following experiment. Drs. H. Gabor and S. Abraham fed laboratory mice diets containing 10 percent fat from corn oil, menhaden fish oil, or hydrogenated cottonseed oil (hydrogen has been added to the molecule to change unsaturated bonds to saturated bonds). Cancer tissue—mammary adenocarcinomas—were transplanted into the mice, and tumors were weighed 21 days later. Tumors in mice fed fish oil or hydrogenated cottonseed oil were 60 percent smaller than those in mice fed corn oil.

The smaller tumor weights were due to increased rate of tumor cell loss, which was 2.5 times greater in mice fed fish oil than in those fed corn oil. The researchers concluded that omega-3 fatty acids contained in fish oils inhibit the stimulation of tumor growth induced by LA by altering prostaglandin synthesis.[33]

Diabetes. It is not surprising that fish oils are beneficial to diabetics because they reduce heart and artery diseases that are associated with diabetes. However, recent research has also shown that fish oil helps non-insulin dependent diabetics (type 2) utilize their own insulin. Type 2 diabetics frequently develop the disease as a result of obesity and their insulin loses some of its effect in controlling blood sugar. Dutch researchers have found that 30 grams of MaxEPA daily improves type 2 diabetics' blood sugar control.[34]

Dr. Margaret J. Albrink, professor of medicine at West Virginia University in Morgantown, examined whether the beneficial cardiovascular effects of fish oils applied to diabetics as well.[35] She found that very large amounts of fish oil (45 milliliters, which contain nearly 18 grams of the omega-3 fatty acids) produced dramatic reductions of blood triglycerides and cholesterol, and returned platelet aggregation to normal without changing the bleeding time.

The above studies are just a sample of the exciting research that indicate there are considerable health benefits to normalizing prostaglandin levels by increasing the amount of fish in our diets. There is also research activity in psoriasis, multiple sclerosis, vision disorders, kidney disease and brain function.

CONCLUSION

Research articles are being published at an ever-increasing rate. The National Institutes of Health are even advertising for researchers to apply for funds to further test and expand our knowledge about EPA. Most scientific publications have now carried news articles and editorials about fish oils, in addition to the research articles they publish. Even the Food and Drug Administration has published a favorable article in its *FDA Consumer* magazine.[36] The health advantages of adding fish oils to the diet are obvious. The question now becomes how to best do this.

Increasing Dietary Fish Oil. It is unlikely that Americans will adopt the Eskimo diet, but there is no need to do so. Having one or two fish servings per week will please many people and convince the skeptics about the taste and meal variety that fish offer. Others may not prefer to do this and will opt to eat more fish on a regular basis and also include fish oil capsules as dietary supplements.

Please keep in mind that deep-frying fish will destroy the EPA and DHA. Broiling is a better method, and many feel that it improves the taste as well.

Table 1 lists the EPA and DHA content of selected foods, while Table 2 gives the total omega-3 fatty acid content of various fish and shellfish. Table 3 shows the amounts of fish, shellfish and supplements which supply one gram of EPA and DHA.

Fish oil supplements are available in a variety of forms, such as salmon oil, MaxEPA, Promega and Proto-Chol.* MaxEPA is a trade name of a blend of fish oils that has been commercially available for some time and has been used extensively in scientific research. MaxEPA is distributed by many supplement companies under their own label. It contains 18 percent EPA and 12 percent DHA. MaxEPA contains no fish liver oil so large amounts can be taken without appreciably increasing body vitamin A and D levels. Promega contains 35 percent EPA and 15 percent DHA.

TABLE 1. EPA and DHA content of selected foods

Food (3.5 oz.)	Fat (grams)	EPA/DHA (grams)	Cholesterol (milligrams)	Calories
Cod	0.7	0.2	37	82 (steamed) 204 (fried)
Flounder	1.0	0.2	46	53 (steamed) 214 (fried)
Salmon	6.6	1.0–1.4	74	199 (steamed)
Trout	3.4	0.5	57	131 (steamed)
Crab	1.3	0.4	78	127 (boiled)
Lobster	0.9	0.2	95	119 (boiled)
Shrimp	1.3	0.2	128	114 (boiled)

Compiled from USDA Handbook No. 8.

*MaxEPA is a trademark of Seven Seas Health Care Ltd., Hull, England; Promega is a trademark of the Parke-Davis Division of Warner-Lambert; Proto-Chol is a trademark of E. R. Squibb & Sons, Inc., Princeton, New Jersey.

TABLE 2. Total omega-3 fatty acid content

Includes shorter chains that may not be converted in the body to EPA or DHA. Some legumes, vegetables, plant oils, nuts and seeds also may contain omega-3 fatty acids, but no study reported to date has shown that consumption of the shorter-chain omega-3 fatty acids such as linolenic acid can produce the physiologic effect of marine omega-3 fatty acids.

Food (3.5 oz.)	Omega-3 (gram)	Total fat (gram)
Salmon, Atlantic	1.4	-
Salmon, Pink	1.0-1.9	5.2
Salmon, Chinook, canned	3.0	16.0
Salmon, sockeye	1.3	8.6
Trout	1.1-2.0	4.5
Sardines	2.9	-
Mackerel	2.2-2.6	9.8-13.9
Herring	1.1-1.7	6.2-9.0
Tuna, canned	1.5-1.7	6.6-6.8
Anchovy	1.4	-
Bluefish	1.2	6.5
Halibut	0.5-0.9	2.0
Sablefish	1.4	13.1
Bass	0.6	2.2
Catfish	0.6	3.6
Perch	0.5	2.5
Haddock	0.2	0.7
Flounder	0.3	1.2
Hake	0.6	2.6
Mullet	1.1	4.4
Pompano	0.6	9.5
Shark	0.5	1.9
Swordfish	0.2	2.1
Oyster	0.4-0.8	2.3-2.5
Crab, Alaska king	0.6	1.6
Crab, blue, canned	0.4-0.5	1.3-1.6
Shrimp	0.3-0.4	1.1-1.2

Compiled from The New England Journal of Medicine 316:625, March 5, 1987.

TABLE 3. Quantities needed to supply 1 gram of EPA and DHA.

Food	Grams	EPA and DHA (grams)	Cholesterol (milligrams)	Calories
Cod	500	1	185	410
				1020
Flounder	500	1	_ 230	265
				1070
Salmon	100	1	74	199
Trout	200	1	114	262
Crab	250	1	195	317
Lobster	500	1	475	595
Shrimp	500	1	640	570
MaxEPA	3	1	14	27
Cod liver oil	5	1	25	45

Compiled from the Journal of the American Dietetic Association *86:788, 1986.*

Some physicians have suggested that vegetable sources of omega-3 fatty acids could be added to the diet, but studies have shown that only EPA and DHA have produced the results discussed in this booklet. ALA is an omega-3, but it cannot be converted in adequate quantities, to EPA, which is needed to form the PG3 family of prostaglandins. Purslane, walnut oil, walnuts, wheat germ oil, canola oil (rapeseed oil that has had the theruic acid removed), soybean lecithin, soybeans and tofu, common beans, butternuts and seaweed are all fine foods, but they are not important sources of EPA and DHA.

A few physicians thought that it was better to have a vegetable source of EPA because fish sources have cholesterol in them. Now this is cholesterol phobia at its best—or is it worst? EPA lowers cholesterol. The same MaxEPA supplements that worry a few anti-cholesterol people are the factors that lowered blood cholesterol levels. It is the blood cholesterol level—and even more important, the ratio of HDL to LDL cholesterol—that is important as a risk factor in heart disease.

A MaxEPA capsule that contains 180 milligrams of EPA and 120 mg of DHA contains only 5 mg of cholesterol,

10 calories, and 50 IU of vitamin A. To get the same amount of EPA from salmon, one would have to eat 30 grams, which would also contain 25 mg of cholesterol (five times that in MaxEPA) and 70 calories (seven times that of MaxEPA).

The safety and benefits have been studied in the articles described in this booklet. It seems to be very wise for the average person to add fish to their diet. However, some people may be allergic to fish or have a medical problem that precludes them from doing this. By all means check with your doctor.

REFERENCES

1. Passwater, R. A. *EPA—Marine Lipids*. New Canaan, Connecticut: Keats Publishing, Inc., 1982.
2. Bennett, A. et al. *Gerontology* 26:74A, 1986.
3. Kinsella, J. E. *Nutr. Today* 7–14, Nov.-Dec., 1986.
4. Von Lossonczy, T. O. et al. Effect of Fish Diet on Serum Lipids in Healthy Human Subjects. *Am. J. Clin. Nutr.* 31:1340–1346, 1978.
5. Van Gent, C. M. et al. Effect on Serum Lipid Levels of W-3 Fatty Acids of Ingesting Fish Oil Concentrate. *The Lancet* 1249–1250, Dec. 8, 1970.
6. Kingsbury, K. J. et al. Effects of Ethyl Arachidonate, Cod Liver Oil and Corn Oil on the Plasma Cholesterol Level. *The Lancet* 739, 1961.
7. Siess, W. et al. Platelet Membrane Fatty Acids, Platelet Aggregation and Thromboxane Formation During Mackerel Diet. *The Lancet* 441–444, March 15, 1980.
8. Harris, W. W. and Connor, W. E. The Effect of Salmon Oil upon Plasma Lipids, Lipoproteins and Triglyceride Clearance. *Trans. Assoc. Amer. Phys.* xciii, 148, 1980.
9. Saynor, R. and Verel, D. Effect of a Fish Oil on Blood Coagulation. *Throm. Harm.* 46(1), 65, July 1981.
10. Lockette, W. E. et al. *Prostaglandins* 24:631–8, Nov. 1982.
11. Terano, T. et al. *Atherosclerosis* 46:321–31, March 1983.
12. Harris, W. S. et al. *Metabolism* 32:179–84, 1983.
13. Harris, W. S. et al. *Metabolism* 33:1016–19, 1984.
14. Phillipson. B. E. et al. *New England J. Med.* 312:1210–16, May 9, 1985.
15. Chochola, M. et al. *Sb Lekar* 87:23–8, 1985.
16. Nestel, P. J. *Am. J. Clin. Nutr.* 43:752–757, 1986.
17. von Schacky, C. et al. *J. Clin. Invest.* 76:1626–31, 1985.
18. Knapp, H. R., et al. *NEJM* 314:937–42, 1986.
19. Kromhout, D., et al. *NEJM.* 312:1205–9, 1985.
20. Shekelle, R. B. et al. *NEJM* 313(13) 820, Sept. 26, 1985.
21. Anon. Nutrition Digest. *Prevention*, p. 100, April 1987.
22. Foley, E. *USA Today*, p. 1, March 4, 1987.
23. Singer, P. et al. *Atherosclerosis* 56:111–18, July 1985.
24. Ibid. 56:223–35, Aug. 1985.
25. Norris, P. G. et al. *British Med. J.* 293:104–5, July 12, 1986.
26. Sperling, R. I. et al. *Arthritis and Rheumatism* 25:133, 1983.
27. Lee, T. H. et al. *NEJM* 312(19) 1217–24, May 9, 1985.

28. Kremer, J. et al. *Clin. Res.* 33:A778, 1985.
29. Glueck, C. J. et al. *Am. J. Clin. Nutr.* In press, 1986.
30. Karmali, R. A. et al. *J. Nat. Cancer Inst.* 73:457–61, Aug. 1984.
31. O'Connor, T. P. et al. *J. Nat. Cancer Inst.* 75(5) 959–62, Nov. 1985.
32. Jurkowski, J. J. and Cave, W. T. *J. Natl. Cancer Inst.* 74:1145–50, May 1985.
33. Gabor, H. and Abraham, S. *J. Nat. Cancer Inst.* 76:1223–29, June 1986.
34. *Netherlands J. Med.* 29(2), 1986.
35. Albrink, M. J. et al. Annual Meeting of the American Diabetes Association, Anaheim, CA, 1986.
36. Zamula, E. *FDA Consumer* 20(8) 6–8, Oct. 1986.

www.ingramcontent.com/pod-product-compliance
Ingram Content Group UK Ltd.
Pitfield, Milton Keynes, MK11 3LW, UK
UKHW021501281225
466417UK00025B/48

9 780879 834326